CARING CONVERSATIONS WITH SENIORS

CHRIS FAIRWEATHER

Published by:
Berhampore Press.
Wellington,
New Zealand.
All rights reserved.
Copyright © 2019

ISBN: 9781089412489

CARING
CONVERSATIONS
WITH SENIORS

Table of Contents

Introduction

This book is simple to use. It contains a series of questions designed to draw out long-forgotten memories and enhance conversation with seniors. These questions will help staff and residents develop trust and empathy for each other.

Ways to use this book:

    1. Use the questions as prompts for day-to-day conversations.

    2. Keep it beside a resident's bed for staff to add information they have discovered.

    3. In cases of dementia, reverse the process and use the questions so visitors and staff can tell stories to the patient.

There is enough space after each question for notes if you want to preserve information.

There are sections about childhood, teenage years, adulthood, parenting, favorite stories and much, much more. You'll be amazed what you discover, and the stories that spring to life.

I hope you find this book as helpful as I have.

Chris Fairweather

A conversation with:_____

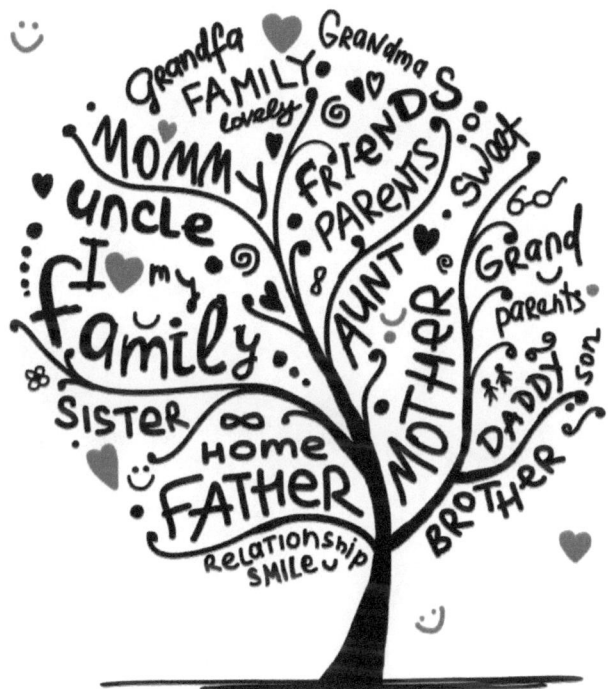

HANDY HINT:

The space after each question is for notes that you may want to keep
for future talks.

Childhood and Family

When and where were you born?

Were you born in a hospital, or was it at home?

Do you know if there were any complications during your birth?

Who were your parents?

What is your family's origin?

What work did your parents do?

What were your siblings like?

How many siblings did you have?

Did you get on with your siblings?

What, if anything, did you argue with your siblings about?

Which sibling did you get on with the best?

What is your first memory?

What do you remember of your early childhood?

Did you have your own bedroom?

What was your bedroom like?

Did your family eat their main meals together?

Did your family go to church, and if so, what was it like?

Were you close to extended family?

How often did you meet up with cousins and other family?

What do you remember about typical family gatherings?

How did you stay connected with other family members?

Did you have a favorite aunt, uncle, grandparent, or cousin?

What was it that made them a favorite?

What is your most memorable family vacation?

What other things did you do for fun?

Who did you play with as a child?

Did you ever have an imaginary friend?

What were your favorite toys or games?

Did you have a favorite stuffed animal?

Did you play any sports as a child?

What do you remember about the house you grew up in?

What could you see out of the windows of your house?

What was your neighborhood like?

What was the city/country like around your home?

How has the place you grew up changed over time?

How far were you allowed to roam on your own?

Do you remember any of the local shops?

What did they sell?

Do you remember any nearby parks or sports grounds?

How did your family celebrate holidays?

How did your family celebrate your birthday?

Do you remember a favorite birthday?

What kind of gifts did you get?

What holiday traditions did your family celebrate as you grew up?

What sort of trouble did you get into as a child?

Were you often punished?

If so, what was a typical punishment and what did you think about it?

What type of school/s did you attend?

What do you remember about your early school years?

Who was your best friend/s at school?

What exciting things do you remember learning as a child?

Did you have a favorite teacher?

If so, what was it that you liked about them?

What were your clothes like as a child?

What did you want to be when you grew up?

Were you ever bullied?

What do you remember about your home life when you were young?

What did you like most about your childhood?

What worried you most as a child?

What things or people scared you as a child?

What were your favorite foods as a child?

What was your favorite time of year?

What books did you read?

What TV shows/movies did you enjoy most?

What were you good at as a child?

What made you unhappy?

What's different about growing up today from when you were a child?

What was your favorite activity with friends?

Were you a member of any clubs or organizations?

What were your hobbies?

What did you collect or obsess over as a child?

What family pets did you have as a child?

Did your family have a garden when you were a child?

Do you remember any of the plants or trees in it?

If you close your eyes, can you picture any of the houses you lived in as a child?

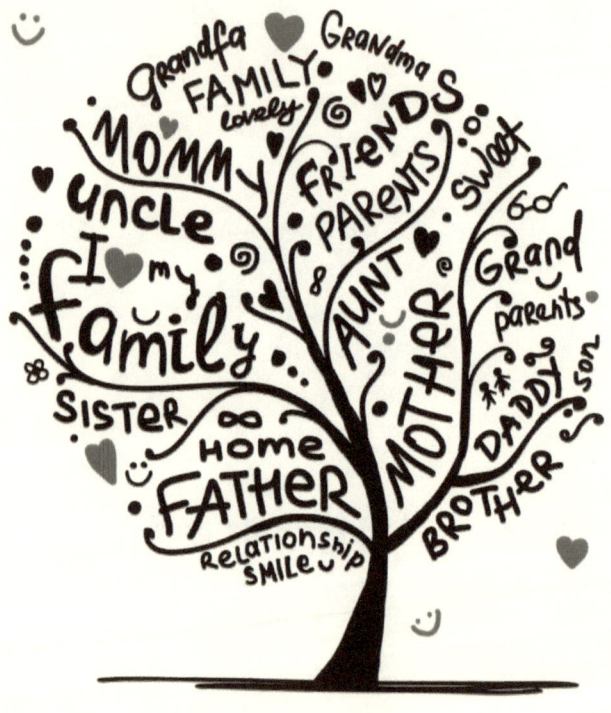

Teenage Years

What was life like for you as a teenager?

Were you an early or a late bloomer?

How did your relationship with your parents change as you got older?

What did you enjoy most about school as a teen?

What did you dislike about school?

What were your favorite subjects?

Did high school help you choose a career?

Did you have a favorite teacher at high school?

If so, what was it about them that you liked or admired?

Did you ever learn another language?

When did you leave school?

Did you feel rich or poor growing up?

Did you ever have to go without?

How did you earn your pocket money?

How old were you when you got your first paid job?

What other jobs did you have as a teen?

Do you remember how much you were paid?

What were the important things you learned while working as a teenager?

Did your wages contribute to the household expenses?

Did you have any favorite clothing or style as a teen?

Where did your clothes come from?

What clubs or groups were you a member of?

What did you enjoy about being a member of a club or organization?

Was there any event/s that shaped the person that you eventually became?

What fun times stand out from your teenage years?

What kind of car/s did your family own?

When did you learn to drive and who was your instructor?

When did you get your first car?

What type of car was it and did you take any memorable trip in it?

What is the fastest you've ever driven and where was it?

Did you go to a church or religious youth group?

If religious, did you ever question your faith?

What did you think about the world as a teenager?

As a teen, did you think the world was a fair place?

If not, what needed changing?

Did you have any goals or dreams as a teen?

How did you want your life to be different from the one your parents lived?

Were you rebellious as a teen?

At what age did your parents start to treat you more like an adult?

When did you first become aware of politics?

What did you worry about as a teenager?

Did you experience racism while a teenager?

What were the big issues going on when you were a teenager?

Did your family have any major issues going on while you were a teen?

What do you remember about your local community while a teen?

Who was your first crush?

Did your parents know/approve?

What was dating like back then?

Who were your musical influences and why?

Did you play a musical instrument or sing?

What were the bands and music that you liked as a teen?

What was the best concert/play/event that you went to?

Did you get involved in politics?

If so, who were the politicians you admired and why?

Did you belong to any environmental groups?

Did you travel to different states or countries as a teen?

If so, what did you learn while travelling?

Did you family move around much while you were young?

Do you have any regrets from your teenage years?

What is your happiest moment as a teenager?

Adulthood

What was your experience when you first moved out of your parents' home?

Where did you go when you first moved out of home?

What were the first challenges you had when living away from your parents?

Did you move from your home town to further your education?

If so, what institution did you attend?

What was life like there?

Did you make any lifetime friends at this stage of your life?

At what point in your life did you first feel like an adult?

When did you first fall in love?

What was your first serious relationship like?

What was it about them that you found attractive?

Do you remember your first kiss?

Did you have an unrequited love?

Were you ever heartbroken?

What did other people expect of you and your life?

Did people expect you to get married and have children?

How did you feel about those expectations?

Did you stay close to your parents as an adult?

What were your parents' political beliefs?

What were your parents' religious beliefs?

Do/did your parents' beliefs coincide with your own?

Did you ever have major disagreements with your parents?

Did you have pets as an adult?

If so, what impact did they have on your life?

Are you a foodie?

Are you a vegetarian or vegan?

Do you have any secret recipes?

Do you like to travel?

What other states/countries have you visited?

Do you prefer planes, trains or automobiles and why?

Did travelling make you re-evaluate your own life or country?

What was your most memorable journey?

What were your impressions of some places you've travelled?

What did you like or dislike about places you visited?

Have you ever been to a casino or racetrack?

Did you follow sports?

If so, what was your favorite team/player and why?

Are you interested in the Arts?

If so, what was the most memorable event you attended?

Have you had any major medical problems?

If so, how did it affect your life?

Were you vaccinated against polio, small pox or other preventable illnesses?

What about the rest of your family, how was their health?

Who were your closest friends?

What did you get up to together?

How did you connect with each other?

What clubs or groups were you a member of?

What did you enjoy about these organizations?

Has military service affected your life in any way?

Have you ever lost a friend or relative due to their military service?

Did you have a main goal in life, and if so, what was it?

What do you consider to be your greatest accomplishments?

How did losing someone close affect you?

What was it like losing parents or a sibling?

What do you think was your biggest mistake in life?

Did you have a particular style when it came to fashion?

Who was your most interesting neighbor?

What was your favorite shop?

What was the best bargain you ever got?

Have you ever been a victim of crime, and if so, how did it make you feel?

Paid and Unpaid Work

Did you have a specific career path in mind?

What was your first job, or volunteer work, as an adult?

What did you learn while working there?

Were people treated the same in the places you worked?

What was your most memorable experience while working?

How many other jobs have you had?

How did you obtain these jobs?

What do you remember about your first pay rise or promotion?

What was your most memorable boss like?

What did a typical day at work involve?

What were your responsibilities?

What did you love or hate about your different jobs?

What were the challenges?

What was stressful about the job?

What interesting people did you meet while working?

Did you make friends at work?

Were you the main organizer at home?

What skills did your various jobs teach you?

Did you feel like your work made a difference?

Were you valued in your employment?

Who did the housework?

What did you do with your money?

How would you describe your working years?

Would you have liked things to have been any different?

Did you do any volunteer work as an adult?

If so, what sort of things did you do?

What were the challenges in that work?

What did you learn from giving your time?

Who were the friends you made from paid and unpaid work?

What's your advice to a young person starting out?

Parenting

What was it like holding your first born for the first time?

When did you decide to become a parent?

What was it like when you first became a parent?

What were the first few days like as a new parent?

Did you know much about children before having your own?

How did your life change when you became a parent?

Did you want your children's lives to be different to your own?

What was the scariest situation you had involving a child?

What changes did you make to your life when you had kids?

What did you worry about most as a parent?

How did you get by financially?

Who took care of the children mostly?

Did you plan your children?

How many children did you want?

Were they any major dramas in your life while you had younger children?

What were your children's first words?

What were some things they did that made you laugh or cry?

What hopes do you have for your children?

What words of advice would you give to parents?

What did you do differently as a parent to your own parents?

What did you do just the same?

If you had it all to do over again, what would you differently?

Did you have any big arguments with your children?

What did your children do that made you proud?

What you like about your grandchildren (if you have any)?

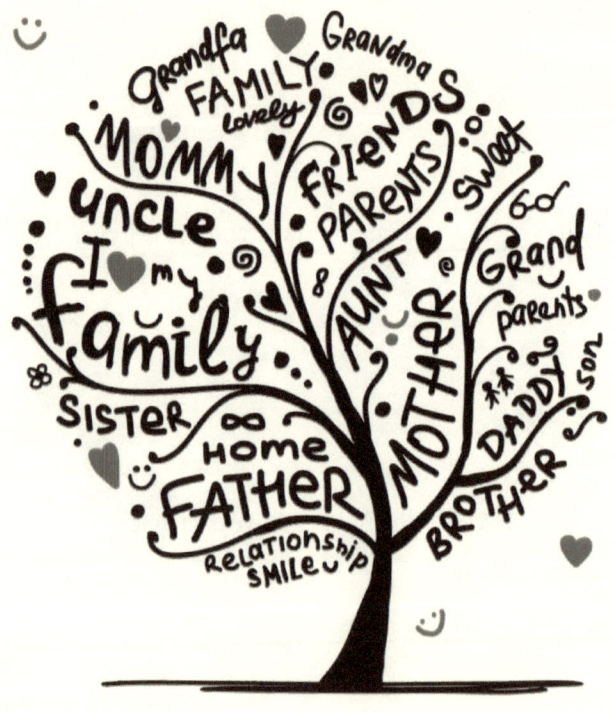

Older and Wiser

What changes have amazed you the most over your lifetime?

What inventions have changed your life?

How do you feel about growing older?

What events have you seen that you thought would never happen?

In what ways has the world changed for the worse?

How would you solve some of the world's current problems?

What issues have become more important as you've grown older?

What problems have been solved?

What issues do think people will face in the years to come?

What sort of world would you like to leave for future generations?

Which things were done better in your day?

What advice would you give to a young person just starting out?

What have you changed your mind about over your life?

What do you now consider the most important things in life?

What are your views on science and technology?

Would you consider yourself liberal or conservative and why?

What are your views on religion?

Have you become more or less religious over your lifetime?

What is your advice about money?

What is your advice about health?

Do you have any advice on relationships?

Do you have any cleaning tips or life hacks?

Which famous people would you like to have dinner with and why?

Do you have a favorite quote?

What genre of music do you like best?

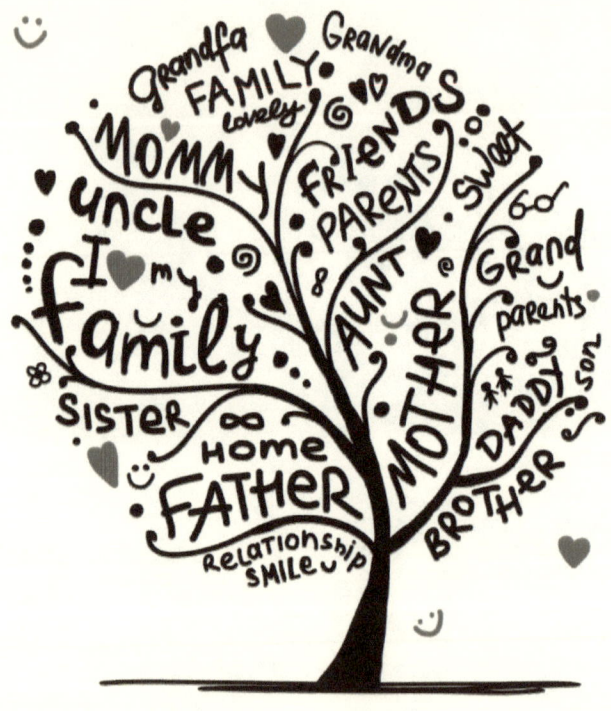

Notes on Strange Stories and Close Calls

Have you ever seen a UFO or other unexplained phenomena?

Have you had any narrow escapes or near death experiences?

What was the strangest thing that ever happened to you?

Was there anything that happened in your life that you didn't expect?

Have you ever had a major fright?

Were you ever in a fight?

Do you have any phobias?

Do you have any superstitions?

Have you ever broken the law?

Did your parents or siblings have any funny quirks?

What are your superpowers?

If abducted by aliens, what would you most like to teach them about earth?

Have you ever seen a ghost?

Did you ever meet your doppelganger (twin from another mother)?

Do you remember any strange dreams you've had?

Have you ever felt an earthquake (and if so how did you feel ?

Do you remember being in a mighty storm?

Have you ever shot at someone/something?

What is the best practical joke you ever played on someone?

What experience would you like to repeat if you had the chance?

Notes on Controversial Topics

(ask/answer these questions with caution, or not at all)

What are your views on sex before marriage?

Do you have any advice about relationships?

What did you do on your first date?

Have you ever had an unusual date?

What are your views on same sex marriage?

What are your views on family planning and abortion?

Do you drink alcohol?

Have you ever have a bad experience with alcohol?

What recreational drugs have you tried and what was that like?

What drugs, if any, do you think should be legalized?

Have you ever smoked cigarettes?

Star Trek, Star Wars or neither?

Is love the answer to the world's problems?

What are your views on the death penalty?

Is war ever justified?

Is torture ever justified?

What are your views on immigration?

What do you think happens when we die?

Are you a dog or a cat person?

What are your views on equity and equality?

How do you think the healthcare industry should be organized?

Do you believe in any conspiracies (9/11, moon landing hoax, JFK etc)?

Do you believe in ghosts?

What are your views on GMOs?

Do you think vaccines should be compulsory?

Should churches be tax exempt?

Are nude beaches okay?

Have you ever skinny-dipped or streaked?

Should the human race try to establish colonies on other planets?

What are your thoughts on gun control?

How far should personal freedoms go?

Do other members of society have rights that may conflict with those freedoms?

Are we on earth for a purpose, and if so, what do you think that is?

Should animals have more rights?

If you are a believer, what is your definition of God?

Do you think artificial intelligence is potentially dangerous?

If you could change one thing about the world we live in, what would it be?

Should politicians have to show the public their tax returns?

Should corporations be allowed to donate to political campaigns?

If you enjoyed the experience of using this book, please leave a review on Amazon. This will help others know if the book is right for them.

Thanks,

Chris

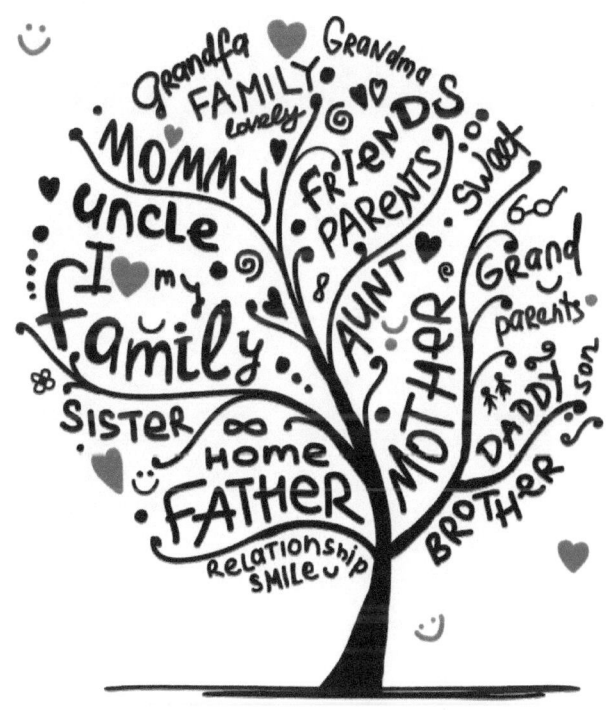

www.ingramcontent.com/pod-product-compliance
Lightning Source LLC
Chambersburg PA
CBHW021236280526
45784CB00005B/2121